Long Distance Healing

Martin Eisen, Ph.D.

Preface

The long distance healing methods discusses in this book are faith, prayer and Qigong healing'. According to traditional Chinese medicine, Qi is the energy which the body requires to function. Gong is the long practice required to control this energy.

Since the concept of Qi is not part of in western medicine, Qigong is defined as a body/mind/breath coordination exercise for purposes of scientific research.

There are various methods of Qi healing. The Qigong doctor first makes a long distance diagnosis of the patient's condition. Then the patient is treated by Qigong methods to correct this condition without contact.

The Qigong doctor can also energize the patient's food, drink or clothes.

Inanimate objects can also be used to help heal the patient

Finally, the doctor can draw Chines characters in the air, surround them with energy, and send them to the patient for healing.

It is hoped that the examples, explanations and research cited in this book will help convince the reader of the plausibility of long distance healing..

Contents

Chapter 1

Faith Healing

This technique is similar to faith healing in the West and involves speaking to the patient. The healing is directly proportional to the Qigong doctor's intention and faith. It is important that the patient have a strong belief in the doctor and feel secure in the surroundings. The stronger the faith of the sufferer and the doctor, the better is the healing.

This method was demonstrated by the famous Qigong Master Shen Chang at a conference of the Chinese Ministry of Broadcast, Film and Television attended by hundreds of attendees. He treated a woman with a three inch tumor on her leg. Master Chang began his Qi transmission and shouted "Gone!". The tumor began to shrink immediately. After he shouted "Gone!" two more times the tumor disappeared completely. To everyone's astonishment he shouted "Grow" and caused the tumor to reappear. After this amazing demonstration, Master Chang made the tumor disappear again and healed the woman.

References

1...Johnson, J. A. Chinese Medical Qigong Therapy. The International Institute of Medical Qigong. Pacific Grove, CA. 2000.

Chapter 2

Healing with Prayers

Zhu You was a minister of Huang Di, the Yellow Emperor of China, and a patriarch of Chinese medicine. He used prayers while doing acupuncture and using herbs to treat diseases. Some scholars believe that he emitted Qi during his prayers. His methods were so effective that according to the Yellow Emperor's Classics most illnesses were treated by Zhu You's methods. Once, professional prayer healers were widespread all over China (1).

In 1993, an Israeli survey of 10,000 civil servants for 26 years found that Orthodox Jews were less likely to die of cardiovascular problems than nonbelievers. A 1995 study from Dartmouth College in Hanover, N.H., followed 250 people after open-heart surgery. It concluded that patients who had religious connections and social support were 12 times less likely to die than those who had none.

Larry Dossey, M.D., co-chair of the Panel on Mind-Body Interventions of the Office of Alternative Medicine at the National Institutes of Health in Washington, D.C., reviewed over 100 clinical trials, in his 1994 book, "Healing Words". Most were published in parapsychological literature on the effects of prayer/visualization. More than half showed a positive effect on everything from seed germination to wound healing.

One of the most widely publicized studies of the effect of intercessory prayer, was conducted by cardiologist Randolph Byrd in 1988. He studied 393 patients admitted to the coronary-care unit at San Francisco General Hospital. Some were prayed for by home-prayer groups, others were not. All the men and women got medical care. In this randomized, double-blind study, neither the doctors and nurses nor the patients knew who would be the object of prayer.

The men and women whose medical care was supplemented with prayer needed fewer drugs and spent less time on ventilators. They also fared better overall than their counterparts who received medical care but nothing more.

In 1998, Dr. Elisabeth Targ and her colleagues at California Pacific Medical Center in San Francisco, conducted a controlled, double-blind study of the effects of prayer, on patients with advanced AIDS. Those patients receiving prayer survived in greater numbers, got sick less often, and recovered faster than those not receiving prayer.

Dr. Matthews is an associate professor of medicine at Georgetown University School of Medicine in Washington, D.C., and senior research fellow at the National Institute for Healthcare Research in Rockville, Maryland. He reviewed more than 200 studies linking religious commitment and health in his1999 book, "The Faith Factor : Proof of the Healing Power of Prayer ".

Dr. Matthews cites studies suggesting that people who pray are less likely to get sick, are more likely to recover from surgery and illness and are better able to cope with their illnesses than people who don't pray. Some evidence indicates that sick people who are prayed for also fare significantly better than those who aren't. In fact, some physicians report that people who are prayed for often do better even if they don't know they're being prayed for.

There are many modern scientific investigations that show the positive effects of prayer for many different medical problems. These prompted Dr. Dossey and several other researchers to state that withholding prayer from an ailing patient is irresponsible!

There are other studies which were not done on humans. If test tube bacteria were prayed for, they tended to grow faster. If seeds were prayed for, they tended to germinate quicker. If wounded mice were prayed for, they tended to heal faster. These studies can be done with great precision. They eliminate all effects of suggestion and positive thinking. Bacteria, seeds and mice and microbes are not likely to be influenced by these factors.

The positive effects, when sick people pray for their own recovery, are easier to explain scientifically. Prayer can be meditative. Meditation has been shown to have many beneficial health effects. For example, meditation inhibits cortisol, epinephrine, and norepinephrine - hormones that flow out of the adrenal glands in response to stress. These fight-or-flight chemicals, released over time can affect the immune system. This increases the odds of developing many illnesses – for example: heart disease, stroke, peptic ulcers, and inflammatory bowel disorder.

References

1...Johnson, J. A. Chinese Medical Qigong Therapy. The International Institute of Medical Qigong. Pacific Grove, CA. 2000.

Chapter 3

Qi in Chinese Medicine

1. What Is Qi? (5)

Before any scientific investigation of Qi, the concept of Qi and its properties in Chinese philosophy must be known, in order to judge how closely any modern scientific interpretation fits.

Qi is a fundamental concept or terminology in traditional Chinese medicine (TCM) with multiple levels of meanings. If you read enough in TCM, you would find that TCM seems to use "qi" to describe almost all invisible forces that affect human lives and health. More specifically, Qi can devote the invisible forces both outside and inside the human body in many different ways (1). We will introduce some of these uses here as we lay out the some basic background of qi in Chinese philosophy and culture.

Qi might have been first discussed by Chinese philosophers (2). *Huai Nan Zi,* a Daoist book around 122 B.C., states that the Dao originated from Emptiness and Emptiness produced the universe. The universe produced Qi,-- Here it was most likely referred to qi energy outside of body.

Zhang Zai (1020-1077) said that the Great Void consists of Qi. Qi condenses to become the myriad of things. He clearly understood the concept of the matter-energy continuum, in the sense of modern physics, even though these ideas were conceived centuries later. He also saw the indestructibility of matter-energy as revealed by his statement "Qi in dispersion is substance and so is it in condensation". Since Qi forms myriad of things implies that Qi must also involve information, in modern terminology. He also said that every birth is a condensation and every death a dispersal of Qi. Thus, just as "Qi" is the energetic foundation of the universe, it is also the physical and spiritual substratum of human life. Zhu Xi (1131-1200) confirmed that Qi condensing can form beings and the conservation of energy, when he stated: "When dispersing Qi makes the Great Void, only regaining its original misty feature, but not perishing; when condensing it becomes the origin of all beings".

From these classic discussions, we should say that a modern scientific explanation of Qi must involve aspects of matter, energy, and information, which remind us of the new finding in physics, the "hidden dimension."

This universal Qi, postulated by Chinese philosophers, will be denoted by "Qi" to differentiate from its usage in Chinese medicine, which will be denoted by *Qi (without quotation).* TCM has been using concept of Qi primarily in two senses. The first use is in abbreviation of functions or conditions. Qi is used to describe the complex of functional activities of any organ. For example, Heart-Qi, is not a refined substance in the Heart, but indicates the complex of the Heart's functional activities, such as, governing the Blood, controlling the Blood vessels, etc. Thus, there is Liver-Qi, Heart-Qi, Lung-Qi, etc. In the sense, it is also used to indicate disorders of the organ's function or body's disorder – for example, "Qi Bi" (Qi constipation) and "Qi Liu" (Qi tumor). These abbreviations will not be discussed in more details here, but Qi as an actual refined substance will.

The second use of Qi is vital energy, which stems from the Chinese character for Qi. Qi can be decomposed into two radicals, which stand for "vapor, steam or gas" and (uncooked) "rice" or grain. In the second case, it is the energy or life-resource within the grain that is called "qi", not the material or chemical part. This is evidence by the fact that rice could lose its taste and "gain qi" after being offered as oblation to the soul. This usage implies that Qi can be used as immaterial as vapor and as dense and material as rice. It also implies that Qi could be just subtle substance (vapor) produced from a coarse one (rice), just as cooking rice produces steam. Thus, sinologists generally agree that Qi is matter-energy in the sense of modern physics.

Natural energies, which are not tangible or visible are particular specializations of this use of "Qi" – for example, Seasonal Qi, Heavenly Qi , Earthly Qi and Food Qi. Other examples are environmental factors or forces that may affect human health, such as cold, dampness, dryness, etc.

Just as "Qi" is the energetic foundation of the universe, it is also the physical and spiritual substratum of human life. In Chinese medicine, the terminology employed depends on the state of the energy-matter. Energetic material, ranging from less dense to denser, is termed: Spirit (Shen), Energy (Qi), Essence (Jing), Blood (Xue), Body Fluids (Jin Ye), Marrow (Sui), and Bone (Gu).

The three most important energetic substances for the function of the body are Jing, Qi and Shen, representing different stages or phases of life phenomenon. These are known as the "Three Treasures" or San Bao.

2. Jing (5)

In order to understand concept of Qi, we need briefly discuss another related TCM concept "Jing". Jing is usually translated as "Essence". The Chinese character implies that it is a refined substance derived from a coarser one. In many senses, Jing could be the internal sources or structure base of Qi. Jing itself can be divided into different types or be looked from different angles. If Qi is used in the sense of function, Jing would be understood as the physiological structure. If Qi is considered as vital energy, then Jing would be the physiological systems that support the energy. For example, endocrine system is frequently referred as "jing" in TCM. Keep it in mind that there are disagreements on what can be called Jing, what cannot. Basically there are three different types of Jing discussed in TCM books.

Prenatal Jing (Pre-Heaven Essence)

At conception, the Prenatal Jing passes from the parents to the embryo. This essence, together with nourishment derived from the Kidneys of the mother, nourishes the embryo and fetus during pregnancy. It is the only kind of essence present in the fetus.

Prenatal Jing determines basic constitution, strength, vitality, and so individual uniqueness. Since Prenatal Jing is inherited from the parents, it is very difficult to influence in later life. Some say the quality and quantity of Prenatal Jing cannot be altered. The way to conserve Prenatal Jing is by striving for balance in all life activities - moderation in diet, work/rest, and sexual activity. Irregularity or excess in these areas wastes Prenatal Jing. Certain exercises help conserve Prenatal Jing, such as Tai Chi and Qigong. Tortoise breathing may positively influence it.

Postnatal Jing (Post-Heaven Essence)

After birth, the infant starts to eat, drink, and breathe on its own. The Spleen and Stomach then extract and refine Qi from the food and drink and the Lung gets Qi from the air. Postnatal Jing is the complex of essences thus refined and extracted. It is the material basis for the functional activity of the body's internal organs and metabolism. The Kidneys store any surplus Jing to be released when required.

Postnatal Jing is continually being used by the body and replenished by food and drink. The Prenatal Jing is enriched and functions optimally only through the action of the Postnatal Jing. Without the function of the Prenatal Jing, the Postnatal Jing cannot be transformed into Qi.

Kidney Jing

Kidney Jing plays important role in physiology. It arises from both Prenatal and Postnatal Jing. Is hereditary, like Prenatal Jing and determines ones constitution. However, it is partly replenished by the Postnatal Jing. Kidney essence is stored in the Kidneys, but has fluid-like nature and circulates all over the body, especially in the Eight Ancestral (Extraordinary) Vessels. Kidney Essence is said to have the following functions:
(i) It is the basis for growth, development, sexual maturation, and reproduction. --- It moves in long, slow developmental cycles (men's Essence flows in 8-year cycles; women's in 7-years) and presides over the major phases of development in life.

In childhood, Kidney Jing controls growth of bones, teeth, hair, brain development and sexual maturation. When Kidney Jing is weak, there may be poor bone and teeth development, stunted growth, and mental retardation.

In puberty, Kidney Jing controls reproductive function and fertility, and normal development into adulthood. Developmental problems that can occur at this time, such as amenorrhea, are often related to weak Kidney Jing.

Conception and pregnancy are guided and controlled by Kidney Jing. When Kidney Jing is weak, signs such as infertility, chronic miscarriage and other such problems may occur. Kidney Jing declines naturally, finally producing the characteristic signs of aging, such as: hair/teeth loss, impairment of memory, etc.

(ii) Kidney Jing is the basis for Kidney Qi --- Jing is fluid-like and therefore more Yin and so can be considered as an aspect of Kidney Yin. It forms the material basis for Kidney Yin to produce of Kidney Qi. Kidney Yin is warmed by Kidney Yang and the heat from the Gate of Vitality

(Ming Men) to produce Kidney Qi. However, Kidney Jing is necessary before this transformation can occur. Kidney Qi can become deficient with age producing signs such as: aching and weakness of the loins and knees, weak bladder, frequent, clear or dripping urination, thin and profuse leukorrhagia..

(iii) Kidney Jing produces Marrow --- Marrow produces bone marrow, the brain, and fills the spinal cord. Marrow in Chinese medicine has no exact equivalent in Western Medicine).
The Brain in TCM is called the "Sea of Marrow". Therefore if Kidney Jing is weak, the brain may be undernourished, leading to poor memory or concentration, dizziness, a feeling of emptiness in the head, etc.

(iv) Kidney Jing determines our Constitution --- Protection from exterior pathogens depends largely on the strength the Defensive (Wei Qi), discussed below. However, the state of Kidney Jing also influences our strength and resistance. If the Essence is "wasted" or poorly stored, the person may have lowered immunity to exogenous pathogenic influences and constantly be ill with colds, allergies, etc.

(v) Essence and Qi are the material foundation for Shen (Mind) --- This postulate is used in Chinese medicine because Jing, Qi and Shen represent three different states of the condensation of "Qi", from coarse, to rarified, to subtle and immaterial, respectively. If Jing and Qi are healthy and plentiful, the Mind will be happy. If both Jing and Qi are deficient, the Mind will suffer.

3. Different Types of Qi (5)

To help students of TCM to understand "qi," modern TCM books started to define different "qi" one way or other. These exploratory definitions discussed below may inspire us to think about the concept of Qi more carefully and comprehensively, they may also create new problem or confusing in understanding the true meaning of qi and its applications in TCM. However, as long as we keep it in mind that qi is more a multi-meaning or multi-component concept than a specific matter, energy or function, we would be less likely to deviate from the original meaning of qi.

Some TCM books have classified the life-force energy according to its location and function in the body (2, 3). Here are some examples of the definitions of various qi for us to start thinking this abstract concept in a more concrete way:

Prenatal Qi (Yuan Qi)

Yuan Qi is said to be Essence in the form of Qi. Yuan Qi has its root in the Kidneys and spread throughout the body by the San Jiao (Triple Burner). It is the foundation of all the Yin and Yang energies of the body. Yuan Qi, like Prenatal Jing, is hereditary, fixed in quantity, but nourished by Postnatal Jing.

Yuan Qi is the dynamic force that motivates the functional activity of internal organs, and is the foundation of vitality. It circulates through the body in the channels, relying on the transporting system of the San Jiao (Triple Burner). It is the basis of Kidney Qi, and dwells between the two Kidneys, at the Gate of Vitality (Ming Men). It facilitates transformation of Qi described below, and participates in producing Blood. It emerges and stays at the 12 Source points.

Center Qi (Zhong Qi)

Energy generated from the Spleen and Stomach, whose function is to transport the Qi from food into the chest where it is combined with the Heart's and Lungs' Qi.

Food Qi (Gu Qi)

Food entering the Stomach is first "rotted and ripened"; then transformed into a usable form by the Spleen. The energy derived from this food essence is divided into Pure Yang Qi and Impure Yin Qi by the Spleen. The Pure Yang Qi is sent upward to the chest by the Center Qi via the Middle Burner. First, it goes to the Lungs where it combines with the Heavenly Qi to form Gathering (Zong) Qi. Then, it is transported to the Heart, where it unites with the Yuan Qi from the Kidneys to produce Blood. The turbid Yin Qi of Gu Qi is sent down by the Spleen via the Middle Burner to the Lower Burner to be further refined and excreted.

Clear Yang Qi (Qing Qi)

This is the pure energy form the Gu Qi sent by the Spleen to the Upper Burner and chest via the Middle Burner.

Turbid Yin Qi (Zhou Qi)

This is the impure energetic essence of Gu Qi transported by the Spleen via the Middle Burner to the Lower Burner to be further refined and excreted.

Gathering Qi (Zong Qi)

This is also called Chest Qi (Xiong Qi), Big Qi Da Qi) and " Big Qi of the Chest". The Spleen sends the pure energetic essence of Gu Qi up to the Lungs, where (with the help of Yuan Qi and Kidney Qi) it combines with air and transforms into Zong Qi.

Zong Qi nourishes the Heart and Lungs. It enhances and promotes the Lungs in controlling Qi and respiration and the Heart's function of governing the Blood and Blood Vessels. If Zong Qi (Gathering Qi) is weak, the extremities, especially the hands, will be weak or cold.
Zong Qi gathers in the throat and influences speech (which is under control of the Heart) and the strength of voice (under control of Lungs). The strength of Zong Qi can also be determined form the voice – weak (strong) voice, weak (strong) Zong Qi. It is easily affected by emotional problems, such as grief and sadness, which disperse the energy in the chest and weaken the Lungs. The Lungs and Kidney mutually assist each other via Zong Qi and Yuan Qi. Zong Qi flows downward to aid the Kidneys while Yuan Qi flows upward to aid in respiration (and the formation of Zong Qi). The chest area where Zong Qi collects is called the "Sea of Qi". Zong Qi and the Sea of Qi are controlled by Shanzhong (Ren-17). Gathering Qi is also treated by the Heart and Lung Channels and breathing exercises.

True Qi (Zhen Qi)
Zong Qi originates in the Lungs. It is transformed into Zhen Qi with the catalytic action of Yuan Qi. Zhen Qi is the last stage in the transformation and refinement of Qi. It is the Qi that

circulates in the channels and also outside the body and nourishes the organs. Zhen Qi has two different forms, Ying Qi and Wei Qi:

Ying Qi (Nutritive Qi)

Ying Qi nourishes the internal organs and the whole body. It spends two hours in each channel, moving through all twelve channels in a twenty four hour period (termed the Horary Cycle). During these periods, the corresponding organs are nourished and maintained by the Ying Qi. It is closely related to Blood, and flows with Blood in the vessels as well in the channels. Ying Qi is the Qi that is activated by insertion of an acupuncture needle. It is closely related to the emotions, since it can be directed by thought.

Wei Qi (Protective Qi)

Wei Qi is fast moving, "slippery" and more Yang than Nutritive Qi. It flows primarily under the skin and in between the muscles, especially in the Tendino-Muscular meridians. Wei Qi protects the body from attack by exogenous pathogenic factors such as, harsh weather conditions, microorganisms, harmful emotions, and evil spiritual forces. For example, a deficiency of Wei Qi can make someone prone to frequent colds.

There are also three Wei Qi energy fields extending several feet from the body. All energetic forms of the body, including organs, blood vessels, nervous system, etc., can be accessed and treated through these fields.

Wei Qi warms, moistens, and aids in nourishing skin and muscles. For example, a person with a deficiency of Defensive Qi will tend to feel easily cold.

Wei Qi adjusts the opening and closing of pores; thus, regulating sweating and the body temperature. It is controlled by the Lungs, which regulates its circulation. The Lungs also disseminate fluids to moisten the skin and muscles. These fluids mix with Wei Qi. Perspiration function depends on the Lungs ability to circulate Wei Qi and fluids to the exterior. A weakness of Lung Qi may cause a weakness of Wei Qi, and lead to susceptibility to frequent colds.

Deficient Wei Qi can lead to spontaneous sweating. When an exogenous pathogen (e.g., Wind-Cold) invades the Exterior, the pathogen can block the pores, inhibiting the function of the Wei Qi, and blocking sweating. The treatment is to restore the Lungs' function of dispersing, strengthen the Wei Qi and produce sweating. Sweating therapy is often used in the early stages of a Wind-Cold pathogenic invasion.

Defensive Qi has its root in the Lower Burner (Kidneys). It is nourished by the Middle Burner (Stomach and Spleen) and is spread outwards by the Upper Burner (Lungs).

Wei Qi has a complex circulation pattern, of 50 cycles during a 24 hour period, 25 times in the day and 25 at night. In the daytime, Wei Qi circulates in the Exterior, but at night it goes into the Interior and circulates in the Yin Organs. From midnight to noon, the Wei Qi is exterior, and is at its maximum strength at noon. From noon to midnight, the Wei Qi gradually withdraws into the Interior, to protect the Yin Organs.

It is said that sleeping under an open window at night gives exogenous pathogens a better chance for attack than during the daytime, since the Exterior of the body is less well protected. Hence, it is easier to catch a cold at night than in the daytime.

Wei Qi can become thicker and extends farther out during Qigong practice. Therefore, it may take longer to move inward at night, causing some Qigong practitioners to have difficulty falling asleep after evening practice.

Upright Qi (Zheng Qi)

Upright Qi is also known as Righteous Qi. This is not another type of Qi but a general term to indicate the various Qi protecting the body from invasion by Xie Qi.

Postnatal Qi (Hou Tian Zhi Qi)

Energy derived from food and drink (from Earth) and air (from Heaven) which are cultivated after birth. Postnatal Qi depends on Prenatal Qi for development. Both form the foundation for the body's vital energy.

Organ Qi (Zang and Fu Qi)

This is the energy responsible for the functioning of the internal organs. The Yang-Fu, hollow bowels, produce Qi and Blood from food and drink. The Yin-Zang, solid viscera, store vital substances.

Each organ has its own energy corresponding to one of the Five-Element energies, which respond to the universal and environmental energy fields. Thinking, feeling, metabolism and hormones can influence the Organ Qi.

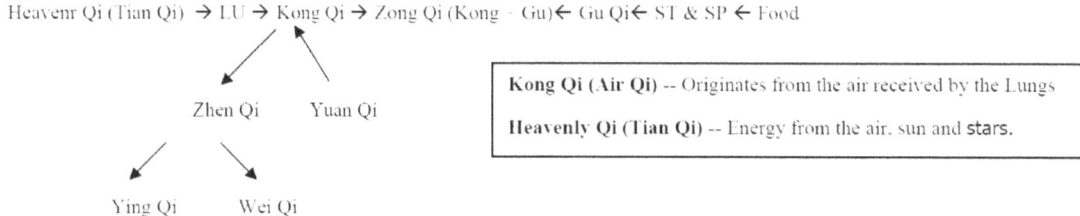

Figure 1   **Production of Wei Qi and Ying Qi**

4. Functions of Qi

The following are seven observed functions of Qi:

Moving --- Produces motion within the body and moves the body.

Transporting --- Spleen Qi transports Food Qi, Lung Qi transports Fluids to the skin, Kidney Qi transports Qi upward, Liver Qi transports Qi in all directions and upward; Lung Qi transports Qi downward.

Transforming ---Kidney and Bladder Qi transform fluids and urine, respectively. Spleen Qi transforms fluids into food Qi, which is transformed into Blood (the Chinese concept discussed below) by Heart Qi.

Holding --- Lung Qi holds sweat. Spleen Qi hold Blood and fluids in the blood vessels. Kidney and Bladder Qi hold urine.

Raising ---Spleen Qi raises the organs.

Protecting --- Lung Qi protects the body from external pathogenic factors.
Warming --- Spleen Qi and, especially, Kidney Qi warm the body.

5. Movement of Qi

The internal organs perform specific functions, normally in relation to a specific type of Qi. In order to perform these functions, the various types of Qi have to flow in appropriate directions. The Liver controls the smooth flow of Qi in all directions. The movement of Qi is based on directions and can be described by: ascending, descending, entering and exiting. Ascending refers to the upward movement of Qi from a lower area; descending means the downward flow of Qi from an upper area. Exiting means the outward movement of Qi, and entering indicates the inward movement of Qi. The following examples illustrate this directional flow.

The Lungs cause the Qi to descend directing it downwards to enter the Kidney and Bladder. The Kidneys receive the Lungs' Qi, while Kidney Qi ascends to the Lungs. The Lungs control exhalation and the Kidneys inhalation. Furthermore, Liver Qi flows upward to help balance the downward flow of Lung Qi. Spleen Qi ascends to the Lungs and Heart, while Stomach Qi descends. Thus, the clear Qi obtained by the transformation of the Spleen ascends and the Stomach sends the unrefined part of the food to the Small Intestine for further processing.

Some organs perform movements in all four directions. Lung Qi moves in and out during breathing. However, when disseminating nutritional essence to the body, Lung Qi ascends, but descends when liquefying waste is to be sent to the Kidneys. Qi exits the Yin organs to flow in the corresponding meridians, while Qi enters the yang organs from their Yang meridians. Qi can also enter and exit the body from acupoints.

Besides the basic four movements, Qi movement is sometimes described as gathering (entering into a location) and dispersing (leaving to a different location). The terms expanding and contracting are also used, but these are just examples of exiting and entering.

6. Qi Pathology

There are four different types:
Deficient Qi --- The Lungs, Spleen and Kidneys are prone to this condition.
Sinking Qi --- Deficient Qi, especially Spleen Qi, can lead to sinking, which can cause prolapsed organs.
Stagnant Qi --- Qi does not move. Liver Qi is susceptible to this condition.
Rebellious Qi --- This occurs when Qi moves in the wrong direction. For example, when Stomach Qi ascends instead of descending, nausea, vomiting, or belching can occur.

7. Blood and Qi

In Chinese medicine Blood (Xue) is not the same as in Western medicine. Of course, Blood is a dense form of "Qi'. However, Blood is derived from Qi in two ways:
(i) Food Qi, produced by the Spleen, is sent upward to Lungs, and Lung Qi pushes it to the Heart, where it is transformed into Blood. The transformation requires the assistance of the Original Qi stored in the Kidneys.
(ii) Kidney Essence produces Marrow, which generates Bone Marrow which also forms Blood.

Note that although Essence plays an important role in the formation of Blood, it is nourished and replenished by the Blood. The blood–forming function of the bone marrow was introduced during the Qing dynasty, before this concept appeared in western physiology!

After a massive loss of Blood, one can develop signs of Qi deficiency, such as, breathlessness, sweating and cold limbs. Qi depletion, such as after heavy, prolonged sweating, can lead to signs of Blood deficiency, such as, palpitations, pallor, numbness and dizziness.

Nutritive Qi is closely related to the Blood and flows with it in the blood vessels and the channels. Four aspects of the close relationship between Blood and Qi are:
(a) Qi generates the Blood (See 7 (i).)
(b) Qi moves the Blood --- This relationship is contained in the sayings "When Qi moves, Blood follows" and "If Qi stagnates, Blood congeals". Lung Qi infuses Qi into the blood vessels to assist the pushing action of the Heart.
(c) Qi holds the Blood --- This action is a function of Spleen Qi. The saying "Qi is the commander of Blood" is often used to summarize the above three aspects.
(d) Blood nourishes Qi --- Qi relies on the Blood for nourishment. Moreover, Blood provides a material and "dense" basis, which prevents Qi from "floating", and giving rise to the symptoms of the disease pattern of Empty-Heat (4). These two aspects are often summarized by the saying "Blood is the mother of Qi".

8. Qi and Body Fluids

Body Fluids in Chinese medicine are called "Jin Ye". The character "Jin" means "moist" or "saliva" and so can be interpreted as anything liquid or fluid. The word "Ye" means fluids of living organisms. There are two types of Body Fluids:

Jin --- These fluids are quick-moving, clear, light, thin and watery, and they circulate in the exterior of the body (skin and muscles) with the Wei Qi. They are controlled by the Lungs, which disseminate them to the skin aided by the Upper Burner, which controls their transformation and movement towards the skin. They moisten and partially nourish skin and muscles. The Jin is manifested as sweat, tears, saliva, mucous and parotid secretions. They are also a component of the fluid part of Blood.

Ye --- These fluids are the more turbid, dense, heavy and slower moving fluids, which circulate in the interior of the body with the Ying (Nutritive) Qi. They are under control of (transformed by) Spleen and Kidneys. They are moved and excreted by Middle and Lower Burners. They lubricate the joint cavities; nourish and lubricate the spinal cord and brain, bone marrow and the "orifices of the sense organs" i.e. eyes, ears, nose and mouth.

Production of Jin Ye (Body Fluids) --- Body Fluids arise from food and drink. They enter the Stomach from which they are transformed and separated into pure and impure parts by the Spleen. The Spleen sends the pure part upward to the Lungs and the impure part downward to the Small Intestines. The Small Intestine separates the impure part into a pure and impure part. The pure part of this second separation goes to the Bladder and the impure part to the Large Intestine, where some of the water is re-absorbed. The Bladder, aided by the Qi from the Kidney, further transforms and separates the fluids it receives into pure and impure parts. The pure part is sent upwards to the exterior of the body, where it forms sweat. The impure part is flows downwards and is transformed into urine. The Lungs disperse part of the pure part to the space under the skin and the remainder down to the Kidneys. The Kidneys vaporize some of the fluids they receive and send it back up to moisten the Lungs.

9. Organs and Transformation and Movement of Qi

Chapter 5 of the book Plain Questions states: "Water and fire are symbols of Yin and Yang." This means that water and fire represent opposite aspects. Based on the properties of water and fire, everything in the natural environment may be classified as either Yin or Yang. Those with the properties of fire, such as heat, movement, brightness, upward and outward direction, excitement and potency, pertain to Yang. Those with the properties of water, such as coldness, stillness, dimness, downward and inward direction, inhibition and weakness, pertain to Yin. Accordingly, within the field of Chinese medicine different functions and properties of the body are classified as either Yin or Yang. For example, the Qi of the body, which has moving and warming functions, is Yang, while the Qi of the body, which has nourishing and cooling functions, is Yin. Yin Qi is sometimes called "Water" and Yang Qi, "Fire". Qi condenses to form the material body and is Yin. When Qi disperses, it moves and is Yang. These Yin and Yang aspects of Qi are the basis of Chinese physiology. The proper transformation of Qi allows birth, movement, growth and reproduction to take place. The movement and transmutation of Qi depend on the function of Chinese organs and will be described below.

The motive force for the transformation of Qi is the Fire stored in the Gate of Vitality or Life Gate (Ming Men), an area between the Kidneys. Historically, the Life Gate's location has been postulated in several different places. Its Fire is referred to as the "Minister Fire'. This Fire supplies heat for all bodily functions and for the Kidney Essence. The Ming Men Fire and the Essence provide another example of the Yin-Yang concept. The Fire depends on the Jing to provide the biological substances for all life processes. Jing relies on the Ming Men Fire for the motive force and heat that transforms and moves the various physiological substances. Without the Ming Men Fire, Jing would be a cold and inert, incapable of nurturing life. This relationship is summarized by the expressions "Qi is transformed into Essence"and "Essence is transformed into Qi". Gathering Qi flows down to the Life Gate to provide Qi and Ming Men Fire flows up to the Lungs to provide heat.

Mutual Assistance of Heart and Kidney

The Heart is in the upper Jiao and corresponds to the element Fire. It is Yang in nature, and relates to movement. The Kidneys are in the lower Jiao and correspond to Water. They are Yin in nature and relate to non-movement. These two elements represent the Yin and Yang of all the organs (Fire and Water). Heart Fire is called Imperial Fire. Heart Yang descends to warm Kidney Yin, Kidney Yin ascends to nourish Heart Yang. The Heart and Kidneys are constantly communicating. If Kidney Yin is deficient it can't rise to nourish the Heart Yin, which leads to hyperactive Heart Fire (insomnia, restlessness, anxiety, flushed cheeks, night sweats, red tongue with no coat and a midline crack). If the Fire of the Heart does not descend to the Kidneys, Heart Heat develops which can damage Kidney Yin and so Water cannot rise. Kidney Yang becomes deficient and edema results. The ascending and descending of Kidney and Heart Qi also affects other organs. If Kidney Yin does not nourish Liver Yin, Liver Qi may ascend too much, causing headaches and irritability. If Heart Qi does not descend, Lung Qi may also fail to descend, causing coughing or asthma. Heart and Kidney Qi provide the Fire and Water necessary for the functions of the Spleen and Stomach in digestion, transformation and transportation.

Spleen and Stomach

Spleen Qi normally ascends to the Heart and Lungs to direct the pure food essence up to these two organs, where it is transformed into Qi and Blood. Stomach Qi normally descends to send the impure part of food, left after the Spleen's transformation, down to the intestines. If Spleen Qi does not rise diarrhea can occur. After some time, Qi and Blood deficiency will occur, since insufficient food essences will be transported to the Lungs and Heart. Prolapse of various organs and hemorrhoids can also ensue, since the rising of Spleen Qi lifts and keeps the organs in place.

Liver and Lungs

Qi flows smoothly when the ascending of Liver Qi and the descending of Lung Qi are balanced. If Liver Qi does not ascend and extend, it can stagnate in may different areas of the body causing feelings of constriction or distention. Stagnate Liver Qi can also invade the Stomach, causing epigastric pain, nausea and vomiting, or the Spleen, causing diarrhea. It can go downwards to the Bladder, resulting in distention of the hypogastrium and slight retention of urine.
Excessive rising of Liver Qi to the head causes headaches and irritability. It can also affect the Lungs preventing Lung Qi from descending, causing coughing or asthma.
If Lung Qi does not descend, fluids will not be carried to the Kidneys and Bladder, resulting in urinary retention or edema of the face. Lung Qi may also stagnate in the chest, causing coughing or asthma.

Transformation of Qi by the Triple Burner (San Jiao)

The Triple Burner is a Yang organ and has been historically defined in several different ways (1). The three divisions of the Triple Burner in the Table 1 are based on the functions of the pertaining organs and not on their location. It ensures the correct movement of all types of Qi. If it malfunctions, Qi, Blood and Fluids will not flow harmoniously and they will overflow, routes will be blocked and Qi will stagnate.

Division	Defining Organs	Qi Function
Upper Burner	Lungs, Heart	Disperses Defensive Qi to skin & muscles
Middle Burner	Stomach, Spleen	Ensures proper digestion & transformation of food it & transportation of Food Qi to Lungs & Heart. It makes sure that Spleen Qi ascends & Stomach Qi descends.
Lower Burner	Liver, Kidneys, Bladder, Intestines	Supervises the transformation, transportation and excretion of wastes. It controls the downward movement of Qi of the Bladder & Intestines

Table 1   **Qi Transformations by San Jiao**

References

1, Wiseman N. English-Chinese Chinese-English Dictionary of Chinese Medicine. Hunan,

China: Hunan Publish of Science and Technology. 1996

2. Maciocia, G. Foundations of Chinese Medicine. Churchill Livingstone, New York, 1989.
3. Johnson, J. A. Chinese Medical Qigong Therapy. International Institute for Medical Qigong, Pacific Grove, 2000
4. Changguo, W., (Compiler). Basic Theory of Traditional Chinese Medicine, Publishing House of Shanghai Univ. of TCM, 2002.
5. Eisen, M. and Chen, K.   Qi in Chinese Medicine. http://yang-sheng.com/?p=194

Chapter 4

Some Modern Scientific Theories of Qi

1. Introduction

Recent scientific discoveries, such as, the theories of strings and subtle energy, can be used to model Qi. Some physical and biological manifestations accompanying Qi in the body, such as, infra-red radiation will be presented in later parts. Finally, effects of external Qi projection on animate and inanimate matter will be discussed.

2. Quantum Field Theory

Quantum field theory was originally created to describe the creation and annihilation of light, because creation and annihilation operations are intrinsically incorporated in each quantum field. Later, it was used to describe the creation and annihilation of sound, electrons and other substances.

The smallest particle of sound energy is called a phonon, which is described in quantum field theory. The idea of the phonon is extremely powerful, and goes beyond our daily understanding of sound. It is essential for the establishment of the field of solid-state physics, which is the basis of semiconductors, transistors and computer chips. For example, the energy of phonons accounts for most of the heat energy of a solid. The warmth of a solid is due to the flow of phonons inside the solid. The interaction of phonons with electrons at low temperature is instrumental to bring about superconductivity as first shown in the Bardeen-Cooper-Schrieffer theory more than 40 years ago.

We cannot see the oscillation of air molecules, but when sound hits our eardrum, we hear the sound. Sound has energy, and carries a type of message to the ear. Sensitive patients can feel Qi moving along the meridians.

Using the analogy between Qi energy and the energy produced by sound vibration, Lo (1) proposed calling the smallest particle of Qi energy a qion. The qion is like a phonon and can be described by quantum field theory. Qions produce oscillations of polarized media in the meridians, which according to Lo are most likely made up of stable water clusters with permanent electric dipole moments. We cannot see the propagation of Qi with our eyes, but when Qi reaches the problem area, infrared image techniques can be used to detect it.

If this theory is correct, coherent infrared radiation should be detected, or even more speculatively, the existence of superconductivity in some state of a human being. Further, in Physics, energy is conserved quantitatively. If Qi is defined in a narrow and precise manner as oscillation on the system of meridians, branches and capillaries, it can be quantified and measurable with detectors. Qi, then, has a strict meaning with precise consequences in that it will be calculated, predicted, and measured by a variety of future instruments. The principle of these instruments is well- known, and used extensively in physics. They need to be modified to apply to human beings. When such instruments are invented and used, Chinese medicine will become more rigorous.

3. String Theory

Many models are possible for any phenomena. The criterion for judging a model is its usefulness for a particular task. For example, a dressmaker's dummy is suitable for fitting dresses. However, it is useless as a crash-test dummy or to construct an artificial hand.

Zhang Zai (1020-1077) said that the Great Void consists of Qi. Qi condenses to become the myriad of things. Thus, to model Qi, taking Zhang Zai's assertion into account, requires that the model of Qi can show that all objects in the physical world can be formed from Qi. Lo's theory of Qi, in Section 2, may prove useful for certain branches of Chinese medicine, like acupuncture. However, it is not the basis of everything. String Theory, discussed below, is a better model.

The name atom comes from the Greek word ἄτομος (atomos) meaning something that cannot be divided further. The concept of an atom as an indivisible component of matter was first proposed by early Greek and Indian scientists. Chemists in the 17th and 18th centuries provided a physical basis for this idea by showing that certain substances (elements) could not be further broken down by chemical means. During the late 19th and early 20th centuries, physicists discovered subatomic components and structure inside the atom, demonstrating that the atom was not indivisible. For example, Rutherford showed that the atom was composed of a nucleus and orbiting electrons. Later physicists showed that the nucleus was composed of neutrons and protons.

An elementary particle or fundamental particle is a particle not known to have substructure – that is, composed of smaller particles. An elementary particle is one of the basic building blocks of the universe from which all other particles are made. Until 1932, the "elementary" particles were the electron, proton, and neutron. Using sophisticated particle accelerators more than 200 subatomic particles have been discovered. However, most are not fundamental and are composed of other, simpler particles (2).

The interactions between the particles are ascribed to the exchange of other particles, called "force carriers". From experiments it is known that there are just four basic forces in nature: electromagnetic, gravitational, weak and strong forces. The last two forces act in the nucleus. The weak nuclear force is responsible for radioactive decay, while the strong force binds protons and neutrons together to make up the nucleus.

The most fundamental theory today that is substantially confirmed by experiment is the "Standard Model" of three interactions: electro-magnetic, weak nuclear and strong nuclear. In this model, particles like electrons, muons, neutrinos and quarks make up matter. They interact via the above forces. The force carriers are other particles, such as photons and the more recently discovered W and Z bosons and gluons.

The Standard Model allows one to calculate the rates at which interactions take place. These rates can be measured in an accelerator or other laboratory equipment and compared with the theory. The result of this comparison has been very successful, and has led to several Nobel Prizes in l.

Today, the consensus is that the Standard Model is approximate and incomplete. It does not incorporate gravity. This is believed to be mediated by the exchange of gravitons, and due to problems of mathematical consistency, no one has ever been able to incorporate gravity into the Standard Model. Another problem with this model is that one has to assume the existence of distinct forces and their carriers. Einstein hoped that there would be a "unified" theory in which all known forces would emerge out of a single one in some way.

The discovery of string theory in the 1970's led to a unified theory. Strings could be closed, like a loop, or open, with two end points. The mathematical equations describing strings allows them to vibrate. Each mode of vibration can be interpreted as a point-like elementary particle, just as the modes of a musical string are perceived as distinct notes.

Some particles, arising as strings' vibrations are very similar to the known matter particles (electrons, muons, neutrinos and quarks). There are others similar to the known force carriers (photons, W and Z bosons and gluons). There is even one particle similar to the graviton, the force carrier of gravity. Thus, string theory produces the known particles and the right types of interactions among them, as in the Standard Model. The inconsistency, which for decades made it impossible to incorporate gravity into quantum theory, has been resolved in string theory.

String theory suffers from some major problems. A physical object or quantity that is a string has not been discovered. As a theory of quantum gravity, it does not yet make any predictions that are currently subject to experimental verification. Another difficulty is that much of theory is still only formulated as a series of perturbations or approximations rather than as an exact solution. Better resolutions of the 10 or 11 dimensions required in string/M- theory and our 4-dimensional world need to be studied further.

Zhang Zai's concept of Qi would be satisfied by equating Qi with the energy of strings. Presently, this would not be a good model to account for the property that the Mind can control Qi. There does not seem to be any definitive research, that the Mind can influence strings.

4. The Field and Mind Intention Experiments

The idea of the zero-point field (4) arises out of quantum physics from the uncertainty principle of W. Heisenberg. This principle states that the products of the standard deviations of the position and the momentum of a particle, such as an electron, is greatert than or equal to half of Plank's constant. Thus, as one of these deviations become small the other must become large. Thus, if a particle was motionless its momentum and positions would both be known precisely and simultaneously, violating the uncertainty principle, since both deviations would be zero..

Adding up all the movement of all the particles of all varieties in the universe, gives a vast inexhaustible energy source in empty space. The idea of a vacuum being simply empty space is no longer valid. If all matter and radiation were extracted from a volume of space, this space is still permeated by the zero-point field with its ceaseless electromagnetic fluctuations. An idea of the magnitude of that power is that the energy in a single cubic yard of 'empty' space is enough to boil all the oceans of the world. "Zero-point" refers to the fact that even though this energy is huge, it is the lowest possible energy state. All other energy is over and above the zero-point state.

In (4), the importance of the Zero Point Field is stated to be that all matter in the universe is interconnected by quantum waves which are spread out through time and space, tying one part of the universe to every other part. This idea might be able to offer a scientific explanation for the belief in a life force or Qi.

Some experiments described in (3) and (4) are that one person's brain waves begin to synchronize with another person's during ESP; exhaustive studies at Princeton have shown that the human mind can also influence REG machines, built to perform a random electronic toss of the coin, so that we can 'will' the machine to produce more heads, say, than tails; human bodies can act as transmitting and receiving antennas; living things demonstrate awareness of the well-being of other living things around them; biofields change when receiving and sending healing intentions; physical health improves when others send focused healing intentions and different forms of meditation produce strikingly different brain waves.

Human beings, on their most fundamental level, are packets of quantum energy constantly exchanging information with the Zero Point Field. However, there seems to be no definitive reasoning showing that the mind can influence small particles or energy in this field, and so large objects

5. Subtle Energy

An eleven dimensional model is used in (6) to describe how the mind can influence the physical world. According to Tiller there are actually two levels of physical reality and not just one. Physical reality is an 8 dimensional space, consisting of ordinary Physical D-Space, with 3 space coordinates and time, and the Conjugate Physical R-Space, consisting of waves described by 4 coordinate wave numbers.

There are two basic kinds of unique substances found in these two levels of physical reality. They appear to interpenetrate each other but, normally, they do not interact with each other, called the uncoupled state of physical reality. In the uncoupled state the normal physical environment can be detected with our five physical senses. But the substance in this normal state of physical reality is not influenced by human intention. The substance in the "new" level of physical reality, R-Space, appears to function in the empty space (zero point field) between the fundamental electric particles that make up our normal electric atoms and molecules. As such, it is currently invisible to us and to our traditional measurement instruments.

The bridge, according to Tiller, is the Deltron. Deltrons are a hypothetical substance which can travel both faster than light and slower than light, and communicate between D and R space. This is of even more interest to us than most particle physics anomalies because Deltrons are, according to this theory, part of the emotional domain. The emotional domain apparently allows human intention to interact with Deltrons, bridging the mind and the physical world. Thus, the concentration of the Deltron and the intensity of human intention must also be specified, which requires 2 more coordinates. Finally, another coordinate is required to specify the intention from the Spirit level. The 11 dimensional model appears in Figure 1 in (6).

The model is formulated using complex mathematics which is not easy to understand by the general reader. The theory predicts that successful "psychoenergetic" experiments occur when there is higher electromagnetic gauge symmetry than usual. Human intention can accomplish this feat, according to the theory, and this allows the novel kind of connectivity between humans and objects that is found in all sorts of paranormal phenomena. Tiller's theory says that human intention can create the conditions for paranormal phenomena because the human subtle energy system (which coincides with the acupuncture meridians and Yogic chakras) actually exists in some sense at the elevated electromagnetic gauge symmetry level.

Tiller invented a device (the IIED) which can measure this critical shift in electromagnetic gauge symmetry and can accept imprints of human intention. The IIED, or "intention imprinting electrical device" is impacted by human intension using deep meditation. This device can then be moved to distant locations and turned on. The activated IIED is permitted to condition a new environment and so affect objects. Tiller has conducted several experiments using the IIED. For example, the pH (or hydrogen ion concentration) in water is affected by this conditioning. The pH can increase or decrease by 1 depending on the intension imprinted on the IIED. Tiller shows that the properly imprinted IIED can influence the activity of the alkaline phosphatase enzyme (ALP) which is a hydrolase responsible for removing phosphates groups from many types of molecules, including, nucleotides, proteins, and alkaloids. Tiller also studies fruit flies; he looks at larval development time, and [ATP]/[ADP] ratios. Again Tiller finds a treatment effects due to IIED, suggesting a direct impact on living organism.

^Tillers model has another interesting consequence. Tiller (7 p. 132) states "Since the reason for inventing string theory was to bypass the mathematical singularity in quantum mechanics and relativity theory so that they could be united, the use of this particular duplex-space reference frame removes the need for string theory when quantum mechanics and relativity theory are mathematically formulated in this particular duplex-space format."

A critical review of Tiller's model by Todd Stark appears in Chapter 9 of (6) and the internet (7).

References

1. Lo, S. Y. The Biophysics Basis for Acupuncture and Health, Dragon Eye Press, 2004.
2. http://particleadventure.org/
3. Green, B. The Elegant Universe, W. W. Norton and Co., 2003.
4. McTaggart, L. The Field Updated Ed: The Quest for the Secret Force of the Universe, Harper Paperbacks, 2008.
5. McTaggart, L. The Intention Experiment: Using Your Thoughts to Change Your Life and the World, Free Press, 2008.

6. Tiller, W. A. Psychoenergetic Science (Paperback), Pavior, 2007.
7. http://www.entelechyjournal.com/toddstark.html

Chapter 5

The Three Dantians

1. Introduction

The ancient Chinese Daoist practitioners described three important energy centers that store and emit energy. These three centers are called the Lower, Middle and Upper Dantians. The character for Dan can be translated as cinnabar or elixir, while Tian means field. Thus, Dantian can be translated as a Field of Cinnabar or Elixir Field. The Three Dantians are strategically positioned along the Taiji Pole. The Taiji Pole is a vertical stream of energy flowing from the top of the head (Baihui point, Du 20) through the center of the body to the base of the perineum (Huiyin point, Ren 1).

The Dantians communicate through the Taiji Pole, which also carries various forms of life energies. At conception the Eternal Soul (Hun) enters the body through the Taiji Pole and departs through it at death. The Taiji Pole also acts as a passageway for the Hun to leave and re-enter the body during life.

The Daoist practiced internal alchemy with the ultimate goal of immortality. To accomplish this transformation, the first step was to gather and transform Jing into Qi in the Lower Dantian. Then, Qi was gathered and transformed into Shen in the Middle Dantian. Next, Shen was transformed into Wuji (the absolute openness of infinite space) in the Upper Dantian. Finally, Wuji was merged into the Dao (divine energy).

The Daoist inner alchemists kept their work secret by pretending that they were actually performing chemical transformations. They used words such as "gold," "lead," and "cinnabar" to describe the supposed chemical reactions for the energetic and spiritual substances within the body.

A chakra (Sanskrit for wheel) is part of the subtle (non-physical) body lying on energy channels called nadi in ancient Indian philosophy. Nadi are channels in the subtle body through which prana, life force or vital energy, which is a non-physical energy, flows. It is an energetic funnel-shaped volume centered about certain acupoints extending to the Taiji Pole. The area around the acupoint on the surface of the body is about the size of a silver dollar. The energy leaves the body through twelve Chakra Gates.

2. The Lower Dantian

Location of Lower Dantian

The Lower Dantian lies inside the lower abdomen around the Taiji Pole. It is a downward trending volume bounded by a downward pointing triangle. This shape allows it to collect energy from the Earth. The limits of its boundary are defined by the three vertices of this triangle, which are called Gates.

The lowest point of the Lower Dantian is the Huiyin (Meeting of Yin) or Ren 1, located in the

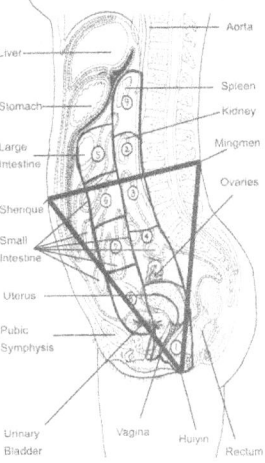

Figure 1   **The Lower Dantian**

perineum, midway between the anus and the root of the scrotum in men, and the anus and the posterior labial commissure in women. A small area, centered at Huiyin, gathers and absorbs Earth energy. This area is responsible for gathering the Yin energy into the body and Lower Dantian area via the three Yin leg Meridians (Liver, Spleen, and Kidney). Ren 1 is also the meeting point of the Governing Vessel, Conception Vessel and Thrusting Channels. This point is also called the Lower Gate of the Lower Dantian or the Bottom Gate of the Taiji Pole.

The Front Gate of the Lower Dantian is the acupoint Shenque (Spirit Gate) or Ren 8, located at the center of the navel. The name refers to the place where the mother's Qi and Shen enter the embryo during fetal development. The small area surrounding Ren 8 is called the Front Dantian.

In ancient China, it was believed that the twisting of the umbilical cord and the internal coiling of the intestines around it followed the patterns of the energetic vortex known as the Taizhong (Supreme Center), which spiraled between Heaven (the head of the fetus) and Earth (the fetus' lower abdomen). It was through the energetic movement of the Taizhong that all things polarized (becoming either Yin or Yang) and received their form. It was also believed that the Heavenly center of this energetic vortex (within the center of the umbilicus) was analogous to the Pole Star in the sky, around which the constellations continually spin. Therefore, the area around the navel was sometimes called Tianshu, the "Pivot of Heaven," or the "Capital of the Spirit."

In Chinese cosmology, Yin and Yang and the three worlds of spirit, energy and matter polarize from the undifferentiated energetic center of the Wuji. As this energetic center begins to polarize, a spinning vortex is created, setting the pattern that forms the energetic template for all things. In ancient Daoism, this energetic interaction set the foundation for the creation of the Prenatal and

Postnatal Bagua (eight trigrams), the original Bagua formations of the Yi Jing, the 64 hexagrams, formed from the 3 trigrams by placing one on top of the other. All phenomena in the universe can be described terms of 64 hexagrams,

Due to this internal connection, the area of the navel is considered to be the home of Qi and Shen, as energetically both Qi and Shen continually spin and manifest from the umbilical area the same way that the stars and constellations spin around the Pole Star. The ancient Daoists considered the umbilical area the "root of preserving life," because Qi and Shen flowed outwards to connect with all of the internal Organs. An ancient Chinese saying states that when the umbilicus opens, the body's internal Organs can interact with the womb of Heaven and Earth.

According to ancient Daoist philosophy, once the umbilical cord is cut, Heaven and Earth separate and the Yin (Earth), Water Qi and Yang (Heaven) Fire Qi of the fetus divide. The Yang Shen rises upward into the chest and Middle Dantian area and becomes the Fire of the Heart; the Yin Jing descends into the lower abdomen and Lower Dantian area and becomes the Water of the Kidneys.

The back area of the Lower Dantian is located at Du 4, the Mingmen (Gate of Life, Fate, or Destiny). Du 4 is located below the spinous process of the second lumbar vertebra. The Mingmen lies between the Kidneys, and in ancient times it was also called the Gate of Destiny, the Mysterious Pass, the Golden Portal, the Door of Fate or the Door of all Hidden Mysteries. It was believed that all of creation passed through this Gate as it emerged from the eternal Dao to form the individual's Taiji Pole upon conception. Physiologically, the ancient Daoists also believed that the spiritual function of the Mingmen empowers the individual with the ability of energetic interpenetration. This ability allows movement within the energetic forms of Yin and Yang, Jing and Shen, as well as the energetic forms of the inner aspects of the early and later Heaven.

In ancient China, the concept of an individual's Virtue (De) and his or her Destiny (Ming) were closely connected. Destiny (associated with the Yuan (Original) Jing, Qi and Shen) was given by Heaven at birth and stored away in the individual's Mingmen area between the Kidneys. The individual's Ming becomes the spark of life and the dynamic potential existing behind his or her thoughts and actions. Although the subtle impulses emanating from the individual's Ming are generally hidden from the conscious mind, through Meditations a deeper realm of understanding can be intuitively discovered and accessed.

Every person must act with his or their Ming throughout life using their Intention (Yi). Their intention is to follow the "Will and Intent of Heaven" (Zhi Yi Tian) to obtai Virtue (De). It is through the development of their Virtue that a person establishes a healthy relationship with the Dao, Heaven and the spiritual world.

The Mingrnen is the root of Yuan (Original) Qi, and therefore determines life and death. The Mingmen provides about one third of the body's "True Fire," supplies the heat for the Triple

Burners, and is responsible for stabilizing the Kidneys and Lower Dantian. The small area centered around Du 4 is called the Back Dantian.

The center or middle of the Lower Dantian refers to its position located between the navel and Mingmen areas. Qigong schools in China differ as to where this center is located. Some say that the center of the Lower Dantian differs because of the different anatomical locations of the male and female reproductive organs. In men, the center of the Lower Dantian is posterior to the Guanyuan (Origin Pass) Ren 4 located on the anterior midline, 3 cun below the umbilicus The center of the Dantian area in a women is higher, posterior to the Qihai (Sea of Qi) Ren 6 located on the anterior midline, 1.5 cun below the umbilicus, within the center of the Bao (Uterus).

Other Qigong schools state that the center of the Lower Dantian is located in the Jing Gong (Essence Palace). The Jing Gong is located at the center of the body posterior to Qugu (Curved Bone) Ren 2 in males and higher in females, posterior to Zhongji (Central Pole) Ren 3.

The Lower Dantian and Jing

The Lower Dantian is associated with the Kidney and is a reservoir for Jing, which is stored in the Jing Gong. The Kidney Jing flows through the body in the Eight Extraordinary Channels. In particular, it circulates in the Governing, Thrusting and Thrusting Channels, which originate in the Lower Dantian. Recall that Kidney Jing is responsible for:
(a) growth, reproduction and development
(b) Marrow production,
(c) basis of constitutional strength;
(d) basis if Kidney Qi.

The Lower Dantian and Qi

The Lower Dantian is also reservoir for heat and energy. It is often called the Sea of Qi because it stores Qi, including Yuan (Prenatal) Qi. Yuan Qi is hereditary, fixed in quantity, but nourished by Postnatal Jing. Some functions of Yuan Qi are:
(a) it motivates the functional activity of the internal Organs, and is the foundation of vitality,
(b) it is the basis of Kidney Qi; dwells between the Kidneys, at the Gate of Vitality,.
(c) it is the spark of change for transforming Zong Qi into Zhen Qi,
(d) it facilitates the transformation of Gu Qi into Blood;
(e) it helps provide body heat.

Yuan Qi flows to all the Organs and Channels via theTriple Burner. It enters the twelve Main Meridians through their Yuan (Source) acupuncture points.

Kidney Jing forms the material basis for Kidney Yin to produce of Kidney Qi. Kidney Yin is warmed by Kidney Yang and the heat from the Gate of Vitality (Ming Men) to produce Kidney Qi.

Since the Lower Dantian stores Qi, it radiates an external field Wei Qi about 1 inch around the body. As the Lower Dantian fills with Qi the field becomes thicker.

The Lower Dantian's Wei Qi Field is the Physical Field. This Field protects the body from the invasion of External Pathogenic Factors (Cold, Damp, Heat or Wind, etc.), interacts with the environmental energies, indicates diseases or future diseases, before they appear. Pathogens can create holes in the Physical Field. If these holes are not treated, it leaves the body vulnerable to attack and disease begins to take root in the body

The Wei Qi Field interacts with the body through its Channels by morphological energetic patterns that assist in the repair of damaged tissues.

Training the Lower Dantian

Nearly all Qigong training begins with focusing the mind and breath on the Lower Dantian. Its purpose of this training is to gather the body's Yuan Qi into the Lower Dantian (called "returning to the source") to strengthen the foundational root of the body's energy.

Qigong practitioners attempt to gather and balance the Yin and Yang energy within the Lower Dantian. This union was called "Dragon and Tiger swirling in the winding river" in ancient China.

Ancient Daoist Qigong, stated that the vital essence spirit always appears inside a bright white light energy in the Lower Dantian.

The Lower Dantian is the closest to Earth and the most Yin of the Dantians. It has the strongest ability to absorb Earth Qi. Qigong practitioners, after having learned to circulate and conserve their own Qi, can increase it by connecting to the unlimited reservoir of Earth Qi.

Everyone's supply of Qi is finite. To heal patients, Qigong doctors extend their Qi and so deplete their own Store of Qi, unless they can simultaneously replenish it from outside sources. If not they absorb Earth Qi. Even people who don't practice Qigong draw Earth Qi into their Lower Dantian as an unconscious action of adjustment to the environment and survival

Qigong students should not attempt to make rapid progress by first concentrating on the Middle or Upper Dantians. Qigong practitioners need the Yin grounding power of Earth Qi to counterbalance the more active Yang energy cultivated during Qigong exercises. Without the grounding in Earth Qi, many Qigong students develop Qi deviations in the form of Excess Heat.

The Lower Dantian and the Mind

The Lower Dantian is the energetic home for the Seven Corporeal Souls, which are collectively known as the Po, and of the Lower Hun, called Yu Jing, or Hidden Essence.

The Po control our survival instinct and the subconscious physical reflexes associated with survival. This is one reason martial artists spend many hours cultivating their Lower Dantians to create the split-second clarity of focus required in life-and-death struggles. The Qi in the Lower Dantian, known as the hara in Japanese, is used for power, stamina and speed.

. This Hun is associated with the Earth, producing our desire for enjoying life and comforts, as well as our ability to fully experience the pure passions of life.

31

The Lower Dantian and Kinesthetic Awareness

Kinesthesia is the sense of awareness of the position and movement of the parts of the body by means of sensory organs (proprioceptors) in the muscles, tendons and joints. The Lower Dantian houses the kinesthetic sense. Kinesthetic communication is the intuition of the physical body. The subconscious mind picks up many signals from the environment that are not processed by the logical mind. The subconscious mind may react to these signals with spontaneous body movements, or with subtle but powerful emotional responses sometimes referred to as "gut feelings."

Often, the feelings experienced in the Lower Dantian are very subtle. Qigong doctors collect energy in the Lower Dantian which increases their awareness and sensitivity. A high level of awareness of the physical body, the surrounding environment, and the relationship between the two, is required in order to maximize kinesthetic communication. When physical awareness is increased, feeling and kinesthetic body movements happen naturally. It is this highly trained kinetic state of awareness that allows the Qigong doctor to feel the patient's internal resonant vibrations. If the doctor's body suddenly feels hot or cold, starts shaking or trembling when examining a patient, this may indicate that the subconscious mind is trying to communicate, and is resonating with the location and condition of the diseased areas within the patient's body..

Another reason that martial artists concentrate on training their Lower Dantian is to increase their kinesthetic sense. It is important to know the positions of their own limbs and also feel their opponent's intensions.

The Lower Dantian and Western Science

The Lower Dantian contains a center of consciousness not in the western brain. According to Dr. Michael Gershon, a professor of anatomy and cellular biology at Columbia Presbyterian Medical Center in New York, the lower abdomen contains the enteric (intestinal) nervous system. His research indicates that the entiric nervous system mirrors the body's central nervous system. It is a network of 100 million neurons (more neurons than the spinal cord), neurotransmitters, and proteins that can act independently of the body's brain and can send messages, learn, remember, and produce feelings.

Dr. Gershon's research showed that major neurotransmitters like serotonin, dopamine, glutamine, norepinephrine, nitric oxide, enkephalins (one type of natural opiate), and benzodiazepines (psychoactive chemicals that relieve anxiety) are active within this enteric system. The enteric system also contains two dozen small brain proteins called neuropeptides. Dr. Gershon's research provides modern scientific verification of the ancient Chinese medical claims that centers of consciousness exist in the body outside of the western brain.

The Lower Dantian can be divided into Nine Chambers each containing a Spirit. Activating the Lower Dantian will result in certain spiritual and energetic awareness (1). The other two Dantians also contain Nine Chambers.

3. The Middle Dantian

Location of the Middle Dantian

The Middle Dantian lies inside the chest around the Taiji Pole. It is an upward and downward trending volume. This shape allows it to collect energy from and transmit energy to the Lower and Upper Dantians. The limits of its boundary are defined by the following six points.

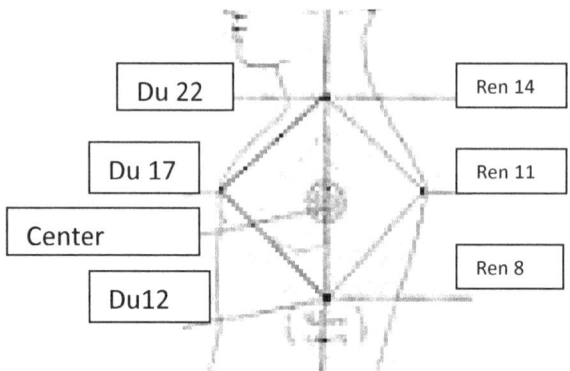

Figure 2   **The Middle Dantian**

The upper front point of the Middle Dantian is located at the Tiantu (Heaven's Chimney) Ren 22. This point is located on the midline, in the center of the suprasternal fossa, 0.5 cun superior to the suprasternal notch. The name refers to the cavity where escaped Heaven Qi from the Lungs pools. It is the intersection point of the Yin Linking Vessel, which influences all the Yin Meridians, and the Conception Vessel. Thus, it is an influential point for accessing the body's Yin Sea of Qi.

The upper back point is Dazhui (Great Hammer) Du 14. This point is located on the midline at the base of the neck, in the depression below the spinous process of the seventh cervical vertebra. It is the intersection point of the body's six Yang hand and foot Meridians and the Governing Channel. Therefore, it is an influential point of the body's Yang Sea of Qi.

The front center point of the Middle Dantian is located at the Shanzhong (Chest Center) Ren 17. This point is located on the midline of the sternum, in a depression level with the junction of the fourth intercostal space and the sternum. A different translation of the name of Ren 17 is Central Altar, which refers to the "place of worship" where the Shen resides.

The back center point of the Middle Dantian is Shendao (Spirit Path) Du 11. This point located on the midline of the upper back, in the depression below the spinous process of the fifth thoracic vertebra.. This point's name is based on to its use as an easy access to the patient's Shen residing in the Heart. It is also the access point to one's moral virtues (associated with the Eternal Soul existing within the Heart), connection to the Dao (Divine) and De (Virtue).

The front lower point of the Middle Dantian is Zhongwan (Central Venter) Ren 12. This point is located on the midline of the abdomen, 4 cun above the umbilicus and midway between the umbilicus and the sternocostal angle. This point is a Hui Meeting Point of the Yang Organs and front Mu Point of the Stomach. It is a crossing point of the Conception Vessel with the Small Intestine, Sanjiao and Stomach Meridians. This energy center is known as the Yellow Court.

The position of the front lower point is debatable and some think it is Ren 15. The location of the Yellow Court is also controversial (1, 2).

The back lower of the Middle Dantian is Jinzhong (Spine Center) Du 6. This point is located on the midline of the back, in the depression below the spinous process of the eleventh thoracic vertebra.

The center of the Middle Dantian is located in the right atrium of the heart, centered between the sinoatrial (SA) node and the atrioventricular (AV) node. The center of the Middle Dantian is considered the seat of all emotions.

The Middle Dantian and Jing

The primary Organ in the Middle Dantian is the Heart. The Heart derives its Yang Fire from the Kidney. To keep the Heart Fire in balance, the Heart also needs Yin. Heart Yin is derived from Kidney Yin. Jing is the material aspect of Kidney Yin.

In TCM, the Heart governs the Blood. Food Essence is extracted from food and drink by the Spleen and Stomach. This Postnatal Jing is transformed into Gu (Food) Qi by the Spleen and is sent upward to the Lungs. The Lungs push it to the Heart, where it is transformed into Blood. The transformation requires the assistance of the Original Qi stored in the Kidneys. Blood is also formed from Kidney Jing. Kidney Jing produces Marrow which generates the Bone Marrow, which contributes to making Blood. Therefore Postnatal Jing, is vital to the Heart's function of governing Blood. Note that Jing and Blood are mutually dependent. Essence is essential for the production of Blood and Blood nourishes and replenishes the Essence.

Middle Dantian and Qi

The Middle Dantian is also considered to be a Sea of Qi or the Upper Sea of Qi. This Qi is Zong Qi (Gathering or Chest Qi). Zong Qi is a form of Postnatal Qi. Zong Qi helps Heart and Lung functions, promoting circulation.

The Zong Qi nourishes both the Heart and Lungs, controls the speech and the strength of the voice, and interacts with the Kidneys to aid in respiration. According to Traditional Chinese Medicine, the Kidneys assist the Lungs in grasping, holding, and stabilizing the breath during inhalation.

Qi and Blood are closely related, Qi is the commander of Blood; Blood is the mother of Qi. Chi Qi gives the Heart and Blood Vessels the strength to circulate Blood, and Qi gives life to the Blood itself. Blood, on the other hand, houses Qi and carries it to all the cells in the body. AQ Blood loss is accompanied by a Qi loss. Thus, Chi (Qi) and Blood are inseparable.

Qi is also inseparable from the mind and spirit. Through the process of refining Qi, the mind and spirit are refined and purified. The Middle Dantian is the main focal point for the refinement of Qi into Shen.

The Middle Dantian also produces an external field of Wei Qi around the body. This field ranges from about two inches to one foot outside the body. As the Middle Dantian fills with Qi, the colors of Middle Dantian's field of Wei Qi change and also become more pronounced. The reason for this change is that the Middle Dantian is connected to the Five Agents (virtues associated with the Five Elements), which in turn govern the five Yin Organs and their emotions. As one begin to experience various stresses and emotional releases, the aura emanating from their internal Organ into the Middle Dantian's Wei Qi field changes its color.

The Middle Dantian's Wei Qi field's is called the Emotional Field, which receives, interprets, and verifies ones emotions, feelings, desires, impulses and thought patterns It protects the body from unwanted emotions, destructive feelings and criticism. It is automatically activated when one is placed in a position where a lack of trust exists, or where there is unwanted physical contact.

The Middle Dantian and the Mind (Shen)

The Middle Dantian refines Qi into Shen and can send Shen to the Upper Dantian. It also houses the Shen and controls all of the functions of Shen that are attributed to the Yin Organs. Hence, the Heart is called the "Heavenly Emperor."

The Heart is related to emotions and feelings in all cultures. All emotions have an effect on the Shen. If the Po, the Seven Corporeal Souls) that are concerned with survival, dominate the Heart, a sense of paranoia is created. This results in a habitual state of worry, fear, sadness, anger, or defensive arrogance. These negative emotions are called "Five Thieves" because chronic states of negative emotions can drain Qi.

The Middle Dantian is the residence of the Middle Hun called Shang Ling (Pleasant Soul). Shang Ling is situated in the Heart and is considered a Soul that is concerned with altruism. It is associated with the Five Virtues and produces the desire to be involved in social activities and responsibilities.

The Hun (the Three Ethereal Souls) control the smooth flow of Qi throughout the body. They are also nourished by the Five Virtues. These Five Virtues give peace and clarity to the Heart and allow the higher qualities of the Yuan Shen to overrule the Po.

An important relationship between the Middle Dantian and Shen is found in the Heart's role of governing the Blood. According to TCM the Shen resides in the Blood and so reaches all parts of the body through the circulation of Blood. This relationship is one reason why anemic patients are often restless and suffer from insomnia. Some forms of unrest can be treated by nourishing the Heart Blood.

The Middle Dantian and Empathetic Awareness

The Middle Dantian houses of emotional (empathic) feeling, communication, and awareness. A Qigong doctor focuses on his Middle Dantian area creating a line of communication with his higher self. Emotional communication is experienced as empathy within the Heart. This empathy is the means by which the Qigong doctor often diagnoses the emotional components of the patient's energetic blocks and imbalances.

All of us are all born with this ability, but as we grow older we tend to ignore this type of emotional communication by depending on the logical mind. Through disuse, this natural empathic ability of communication is lost. The disconnection from this higher perception is the result of the negative messages received from parents and society. Empathetic awareness can be regained by reconnecting with the intuitive self by looking inward and becoming one with the true self that is connected to the divine.

The Pericardium, called the Minister of Council and the Heart's Protector, stores emotional experiences that the Heart was not yet ready to process in the Yellow Court. These emotions would stay outside the Heart in the Yellow Court until the Heart was ready to face them.

Training the Middle Dantian

Medical Qigong students learn to focus their mind and breath on the Middle Dantian to regulate the Heart. Deficient conditions are treated by sending Qi into the Heart and Middle Dantian area, and then regulating the body's energetic fields. Excess conditions are treated by leading the Excess Qi from the Heart and Middle Dantian areas and releasing it outward through the body's extremities.

Medical Qigong students also focus on the Middle Dantian in order to release their own psycho-emotional patterns. After sufficient development of the Middle Dantian, the student will have the sensitivity to correctly diagnose the patient's psycho-emotional patterns.

Medical Chi Kung practitioners strive to gather and balance both the Yin and Yang energy within the Middle Dantian. In TCM the union of Yin and Yang energy within the Middle Dantian was called, "The Sun and Moon reflecting on each other in the Yellow Palace." The ancient Daoist Qigong practitioners believed that the "spirit of man," who stands as a liaison spirit between Heaven and Earth, always appears in a golden yellow light energy, and resides within the Middle Dantian.

Ancient Daoist Qigong masters thought that it was harmful for women to focus on their Lower Dantian for lengthy time periods, especially during menses. The Treatise of Spiritual Alchemy for Women states that the Lower Dantian was considered to be an area for women to focus on only in the beginning stages of their practice. First they should complete the Microcosmic and Macrocosmic Orbit (connecting the Qi of the Governing and Conception Channels with the extremities) meditations. Then, women should focus their attention on the Middle Dantian, As the collected energy in their Middle Dantian overflows, it moves into their breasts, causing their nipples to become erect, and opening one hundred energy channels within their bodies.

Middle Dantian and Western Science.

The thymus gland is located in the Middle Dantian. In children, the thymus gland is quite large but shrinks with maturity. However, scientists discovered that the thymus gland plays a major role in maturing the white blood cells to become immunocompetent and its function continues throughout one's life.

The same neurotransmitters and biochemical constituents that are linked to consciousness are synthesized and created by the white blood cells (3). Therefore, not only do the brain and abdomen have their own consciousness and nervous systems, but the Blood does as well. Hence. consciousness is possible anywhere in the body via the Shen, which resides in the Blood. This was a postulate of TCM for thousands of years.

The heart retains memory and the emotion of love as shown by the following facts (4). Children who had heart transplants and did not know the donors or the donors' parents knew the parents when they met them. Further, they exhibited love to the donors' parents and some characteristics of the donors. A man on a heart/lung machine said he felt no love for his grandchildren while on the machine.

The Middle Dantian can also be divided into nine Chambers (1, 2).

4. The Upper Dantian

The Upper Dantian collects Heaven's Qi and represents the spiritual aspect of man and his connection to the divine. It is also the house of spiritual (intuitive) communication, awareness, and feelings. This is where Shen or spirit is refined into Wu Wei or emptiness.

Location of the Upper Dantian

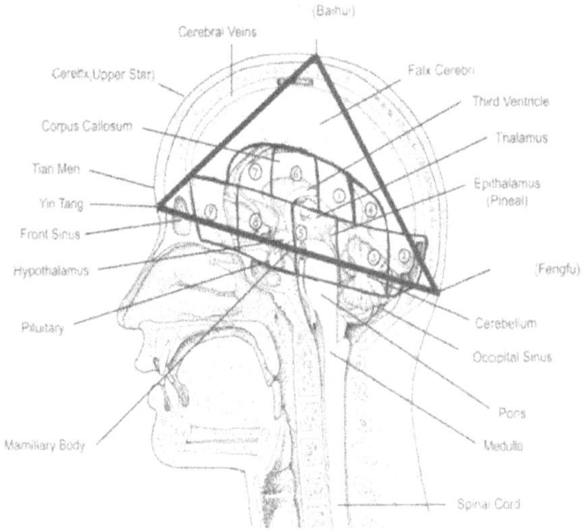

Figure 3   **The Upper Dantian**

The Upper Dantian is centered in the head, approximately three inches posterior to the center of the eyebrows. Its volume is shaped like an upright pyramid, for ease in gathering Heaven's energy. The boundaries of its volume are determined by three points.

The front lower point of the Upper Dantian is the Extra Point Yintang (Hall of Impression) also called Seal Hall or Seal Mark. It is located at the glabella, on the midpoint between the medial extremities of the eyebrows. The name refers to the ancient Buddhist tradition of putting a red mark over this Hall to mark its location as a Third Eye. When the Third Eye opens the Upper Dantian is flooded with spiritual light.

The back lower point of the Upper Dantian is Fengfu (Wind Mansion) Du 16. This point is located on the midline at the nape of the neck, in the depression immediately below the external occipital protuberance, between m. trapezius on both sides.

This area is also connected with the Tianzhu (Celestial Pillar) B 10 points. B 10 is located 1.3 cun lateral to the midpoint of the posterior hairline and in the depression on the lateral aspect of m. trapezius. These points act like an antenna for receiving messages. Qigong doctors enter a trance and receive messages from spirits who extend their Qi and Shen into the doctors' body through the B 10 points.

B 10 is a Sea of Marrow acupoint used to affect the flow of Qi and Blood to the Brain. It is also a Window of Heaven Point (one of eleven acupoints used for treating Shen disturbances). In addition, B10 is one of the Thirteen Ghost Points (used for treating spirit possession) identified by the ancient TCM doctor Sun Simiao. Medical Qigong teachers have observed that students with a more prominent occipital protuberance tend to see auras more easily and develop psychic intuition faster.

The highest point of the Upper Dantian is the Baihui (Humdred Convergence) Du 20. This point is located on the midline of the head, 5 cun directly above the midpoint of the anterior hairline, approximately on the midpoint of the line connecting the apices of both ears. The name, "Baihui" refers to the ancient understanding that an individual can access and receive divine messages and spiritual intuitions through this point. The ancient Daoists thought that the Baihui is one of the areas that direct the Heavenly Qi into the Chamber of Mysterious Elixir, located within the third ventricle of the Brain. The Baihui is the upper gate of the Taiji Pole.

The Upper Dantian is located in the center of the Brain, in an area that contains the pineal, pituitary, thalamus, and hypothalamus glands.

This area is also thought to be the space where the Shen merges with Wuji, the infinite space the formless void. From the Wuji, the Shen evolves towards reuniting with the Dao.

The Upper Dantian and Jing

The Brain, one of the six Extraordinary Organs, is the chief Organ of the Upper Dantian. Recall that Kidney Jing the basis for Marrow and Bone Marrow. The Brain is a form of Marrow and so is called the Sea of Marrow.

Jing and Qi form the material foundation for Shen. Shen is used to denote the close relationship between the mind and spirit, even in modern Chinese medicine.

The term Prenatal Wu Jing Shen is used in Medical Qigong to describe the body's Original Five Essence Spirits (Hun, Po, Zhi, Yi, and Shen). These Spirits combine the energetic essence of the five Yin Organs to create the body's innate spiritual consciousness.

Some styles of Qigong conserve Jing and send its energy from the Lower Dantian through the Taiji Pole to nourish the Brain. Such nourishment benefits the mind and enhances spiritual consciousness.

The Upper Dantian and Qi

The head is the most Yang part of the body and closest to heaven. The Qi in the Upper Dantian is Yang in nature. The Spleen and Kidneys send the Clear Yang Qi which is pure, light, and insubstantial, upwards to the Brain to facilitate mental clarity and activity.

Heavenly Qi is absorbed through the highest point, the Baihui, of the Upper Dantian. This Qi is the Qi from the sun, moon, planets, and stars. It is directed into the Chamber of Mysterious Elixir, located within the third ventricle of the Brain.

The Wei Qi field of the Upper Dantian extends a few feet to several hundred yards depending on the person's spiritual evolution. The dominant color of the aura surrounding the Qigong practitioner depends on which of the Dantians is dominant. The most powerful healers are considered to be those in which the Upper Dantian is dominant and the color will be white.

The Upper Dantian's Wei Qi Field is called the Spiritual Field. It is associated with intuition, inspiration, creativity and visionary insights. It is responsible for establishing security by intuitively informing the body of impending encounters, conflicts or transitions. It receives subtle energy of the finest and fastest vibrations. It senses and interprets the data received from its intuitive environmental awareness and universal connection to the Dao.

The Upper Dantian and Shen

The Upper Dantian is the place where the Eternal Soul connects with the Wuji and then with the Dao. The awareness associated with this union surpasses conceptual thought and words.

The Upper Dantian houses the Upper Hun called Tai Guang or Eminent Light. This Hun connects with Heaven striving for physical, mental, emotional, and spiritual purity.

The Shen can both exit and enter the body from the Upper Dantian by way of the Baihui, Yin Tang, or Tian Men Heavenly Gate) points (defined below in Training of Upper Dantian).

The Upper Dantian and Spiritual Awareness

Five spiritual principles must be ingrained before communication between the individual and the higher self becomes fully open and operates on demand. These spiritual principles are:
(a) purity of intention,
(b) no hidden agendas,
(c) surrender to the Divine Will,
(d) believe and expects success;
(e) have a quiet and receptive stillness of mind.

Communication with the higher self may occur infrequently even after many years of practice. Strong faith is required to open this line of communication. Logic cannot build faith. The Qigong student should not give up. Through dedicated practice faith is established, because communication with the higher self becomes more frequent.

Qigong students must be able to distinguish between true and false messages reflected through their visions. True visions are received from the divine connection to the Dao or Wuji. False visions reflect messages from the subconscious.

Although intuitive communication from within is usually felt as a strong impulse, the Qigong student must learn to keep the logical mind from interfering by practicing spiritual meditations. These meditations involve establishing and strengthening clear links of communication with the higher self. They should be practiced repeatedly until this connection becomes a natural, recurring phenomenon, The more one practices using the five spiritual principles and stilling the logical mind, the easier it becomes to receive a clear communication from the higher self.

Training the Upper Dantian

In Medical Qigong training of the Upper Dantian is for cultivating spiritual intuition.. Upper Dantian training exercises are known as Shengong meditations. These are the major methods used for enhancing the doctor's psychic ability.

The Chi Kung doctor may absorb universal and environmental Qi into the Upper Dantian through the Baihui, Yin Tang (Third Eye region), and the Heaven's Gate or Tian Men (line located in the center of the forehead from Yin Tang to Baihui) points. The energy is gathered and then directed as healing energy to the patient through either the Yin Tang or Tian Men points. \

The Upper Dantian can be divided into nine Chambers or Palaces. The Gates or acupoints that influence each Palace lie on the Tian Men line. The Palaces and their Gates are:
1. Mingtanggong (Light Hall Palace, Courtyard Palace) whose Gate is 1 cun above Yintang
2. Dongfanggong (Cavern Chamber Palace) whose Gate is 2 cun above Yintang.
3. Niwangong (Muddy Pellet or Clay Ball Palace) whose Gate is 3 cun above Yintang.
4. Liuzhugong (Flowing Pearl Palace) whose Gate is 4 cun above Yintang as is Du 23.
5. Yudigong (Jade Emperor Palace) whose Gate is 5 cun above Yintang as is Du 22.
6. Jizhengong (Ultimate Reality Palace) whose Gate is 6 cun above Yintang.
7. Tiantinggong (Celestial Courtyard Palace) whose Gate is 2 cun above Yintang.
8. Xuandangong (Mysterious / Dark Cinnabar Palace) whose Gate is 4 cun above Yintang as is Du 23.
9. (Taihuanggong (Great Sovereign Palace) whose Gate is 5 cun above Yintang as Du 22.

Niwan is used to denote the whole Upper Dantism as well as one of the nine Palaces.

Medical Chi Kung practitioners strive to gather and balance Yin and Yang energy within the Upper Dantian and ultimately achieve Embryonic Breathing (6). Embryonic or Primordial Breathing is to allow the breathing to become effortless, slowed down and may even stop A feather held under the nose will not move. Qi enters the body during inhalation but does not leave during exhalation. You will be lead into a state of blissful stillness and feel like you are unified with the Dao. After this meditation, your mind and body will feel as if you have recaptured the vitality of a child.

Some ancient Daoist sects believed that when Embryonic Breathing was accomplished, a blue-green light energy appeared as a luminous mist within the Niwan Palace of the Upper Dantian.

Some Daoist Masters stated that when one reached an advanced stage of internal cultivation, e, the inner apertures of the Upper Dantian's Nine Chambers would open. This would reveal nine small circular spheres revolving around a large sphere of light. This large sphere corresponds to the sun and the nine smaller light spheres correspond to the nine planets, like in our solar system (2).

The Upper Dantian and Western Science

Recall that the Upper Dantian is centered in the brain.   Some Western scientific information about the brain appears in section 10.3.

The brain receives, reacts to and generates electrical, light and magnetic energy. The function of the Brain is dependent on the interactions of countless energetic structures within these fields. These particular forms of energy stimulate the pineal, pituitary, thalamus, and hypothalamus glands, influencing mental and emotional states. The brain is also influenced by heat and sound, but does not use or generate them to the degree that it generates light, electricity, and magnetism.

The pineal gland, which is a small, reddish-gray colored gland attached to the base of the third ventricle of the brain, in front of the cerebellum. It contains corpuscles resembling nerve cells and small hard masses of calcareous particles. The pineal is larger in children than in adults and more developed in women than in men. Thinking produces vibrations within the surrounding energy field and is radiated from the body as electromagnetic waves and pulses. The pineal gland receives impressions through these vibrations caused by thoughts produce by thinking. Some consider it to be the organ of telepathic communication,

Both the pineal gland and hypothalamus have been shown to be extremely sensitive to light. Dr. Becker (7) cites experiments with bees and species of birds that navigate by sunlight. These birds have disproportionately large pineal glands, which might account for this ability. Dr. Becker also observed that birds seem to have a second navigation system based upon their sensitivity to the Earth's electromagnetic field.

References

1. Johnson, J.A. Chinese Medical Qigong Therapy. Int. Institute of Medical Qigong, Pacific Grove, CA, 2000.
2. Johnson, J.A. Dantians. http://www.ichikung.com/html/dantians.php
3. Candace, P. Molecules of Emotion: The Science Behind Mind-Body Medicine, Simon & Schuster, New York, NY, 1999.
4. Keown, D. The Spark in the Machine. Singing Dragon, Philadelphia, Pa, 2014.
5. Pregadio, F., ed. The Encyclopedia of Taoism. Routledge (2 vol.). Milton Park Abingdon, OX14 4RN, 2013.
6. Cohen, K. The Way of Qigong The Art and Science of Chinese Energy Healing. Ballatine Books, New York, NY, 1997.
7. Becker, R.O.,Selden, G. The Body Electric. Morrow, New York, 1985.

Chapter 6

Two Famous Qigong Teachers Experiences with Remote Healing

Dr. Johnson states that he did not believe in Long Distance Qi Healing (1). One day, one of his Medical Qigong teachers called him. As they were conversing, he felt searing heat in his lower back around the Kidneys and Mingmen areas. His instructor explained that she was holding a pillow, which represented his body, and was treating his Kidneys with her right hand. He said he had no prior knowledge of this treatment or had he given any consent. After that, his attitude changed and he began to study Long Distance Qi Healing.

In (2), Kenneth Cohen tells the following story. His teacher, Dr. Wong, had a very successful Chinese medical practice. Often, he had too many patients with serious conditions and so could not give them timely appointments. He invited the patients to dine with him and did remote healings. After dining with Dr. Wong, most of his patients cancelled their appointments, since they felt better.

References

1. Johnson, J. A. Chinese Medical Qigong Therapy. The International Institute of Medical Qigong, Pacific Grove, CA, 2000.

2. Cohen, K.S. The Way of Qigong. Ballantine Books, New York, 1997

Chapter 7

Remote Healing

1. Long Distance Healing Method Effects According to Tiller's Theory (1, 3)

Different Qigong schools have various Long Distance Healing techniques. This method requires the Qi in the Middle and Lower Dantians to overflow and to transform into Shen. Then, the Shen is united with Heavenly Qi and extended outside the body.. This energy can instantly cross space and so allowing the Qigong doctor to treat patients without physical contact.

The first step is to use your intention to connect all three Dantians by absorbing Heavenly Qi into the Taiji Pole (the center core of light which joins the body's three Dantians and the Eternal Spirit). This procedure is called the "empowerment with divine Qi" or the "hookup". It causes the doctor's Wei Qi Field to be surrounded with Tian Qi (Heavenly Energy), which is consequently changed into Tian Shen (Heavenly Spirit). Then, you visualize a stream of white light emanating from the Yin Tang (Third Eye) point to the patient's body. Once you feel this connection the treatment can begin.

Before treating the patient, you must make a diagnosis by using long distance scanning. This ability can be developed after a few months of practice as follows. Have a patient sit in front of you, close your eyes and perform the hookup. Try to imagine the patient's internal and external energetic body just as if you were making a Qigong diagnosis with your eyes open. Then, open your eyes and perform your usual Qigong diagnosis. Continue practicing until your long distance scanning abilities become very accurate.

After the diagnosis, the doctor uses long distance Dispersing (the spreading of Qi to other parts of the body or purging of pathogenic energy from the body) or adds energy to the body or both.

To accomplish long distance Dispersing, the doctor hookups with the patient and imagines his body enclosed in a ball of brilliant, white light. Then, the doctor sends this light from the top of his head to the top of the patient's head to envelop the patient's whole body. The doctor visualizes this light energy descending down the patient's body and carrying the patient's diseased energy into the ground. The patient's pathogenic energy is sent to the Earth's core fire and then sent back to the patient as pure, refined Earth Qi. Next, the doctor focuses on areas of the patient's requiring attention. These areas appear dark and the doctor imagines these areas becoming lighter. After all the dark areas are dispersed and become lighter, the doctor must disconnect from the patient's body and withdraw his projected Shen back into his own body.

Before sending healing energy to a patient, the doctor stores Heavenly Qi in his lower Dantian and Taiji Pole. To accomplish this, the doctor sits on the edge of a chair with his feet flat on the floor with both palms facing each other at throat level. The middle fingers are pointing straight up and he visualizes a ball of white energy between his palms. He pulls Heavenly Qi to the center of the ball through his fingers. After the ball is completely filled, he imagines the excess Qi flowing into the Laogong Points and descending down the arms and Taiji Pole to collect in the lower Dantian and Kidney areas. Then, the doctor imagines the patient in the center of the ball. However, instead of allowing the excess energy to overflow into his palms, he focuses this energy into the patient's body to fill and cleanse it and so heal the illness.

2. Using Inanimate Objects to Heal Distant Patients (1)

Objects like a pillow or an acupuncture model are used. The doctor places the object, for example - a doll, on a table in front of him. He draws the Essence of the patient into the doll. Then, the patient is treated by removing the pathogenic energy from the doll. When the Qigong master feels that the distant patient has been sufficiently cleansed and the illness dispersed, he tonifies the patient's weak organs through their representation in the doll. You can feel hot and colds spots at acupuncture points on the treated doll.

3. Using Items Made or Worn by a Patient for Treatment (1)

Dr. Johnson describes the following experience, which occurred at the Third World Medical Conference on Medical Qigong in Beijing, China in 1996. He was sketching while listening to a lecture. A Qigong Master noticed my artwork and asked to see it. He placed his hand above the picture and began to project Qi into the drawing. Immediately Dr. Johnson's felt that his whole body was filled with light and sound and he began to vibrate all over. Since Dr. Johnson's art was connected to his physical energy, the Master was able to project energy into Dr. Johnson's body by projecting energy into Dr. Johnson's drawings.

Art or any object touched or created by a person is imprinted with the person's unique, encoded energy pattern. Using psychometry (the art of sensing thoughts, images, etc. which an object has been imprinted), a connection to the person who held or created the object can be created. Using his intent, the doctor can use this object as a focusing point to send healing energy the owner of the object.

4. Healing by Projecting Chinese Characters (1)

Another method a Qigong doctor uses to heal is by drawing Chinese Characters in the air, surrounding them by a brilliant ball of white light energy and sending them into the patient's body. The doctor's intention creates the projected energy. The patient's desire to heal creates a receptive attitude to absorb the projected energy.

5. Healing by Energizing Material, Liquid or Food (1)

Some Qigong doctors energize paper or cloth, which is placed on the patient or worn, to produce healing. Others energize liquids for healing, such as: wines, herbal teas, IV fluids or simply water. These doctors send the energized liquids to their patients, who ingest them to tonify their deficiencies. Plain water is an excellent energy carrier, since it can absorb many different electromagnetic vibrations. Other Qigong doctors energize food before it is eaten by the patient, because ingested food is transformed by the body into energy (Gu Qi).

6. Healing Using Crystals (1)

Some crystals emit a very strong white light energy. These can be used for cutting pathogenic Qi from a patient's tissues and cleansing the patient by scooping out energetic toxins. They can also remove pathogenic Qi from the patient's external Qi field.

Crystals can enhance the Qigong doctor's projection and energetic extension abilities and so improve tonification.

References

1. Johnson, J. A. Chinese Medical Qigong Therapy. The International Institute of Medical Qigong, Pacific Grove, CA, 2000.

2. Cohen, K.S. The Way of Qigong. Ballantine Books, New York, 1997.

3. Tiller, W. A. Psychoenergetic Science (Paperback), Pavior, 2007.

4. http://www.entelechyjournal.com/toddstark.html